KIDNEY-FRIENDLY VEGAN COOKBOOKS

Delicious Vegan Recipes for Kidney Health

T. John

COPYRIGHT PAGE

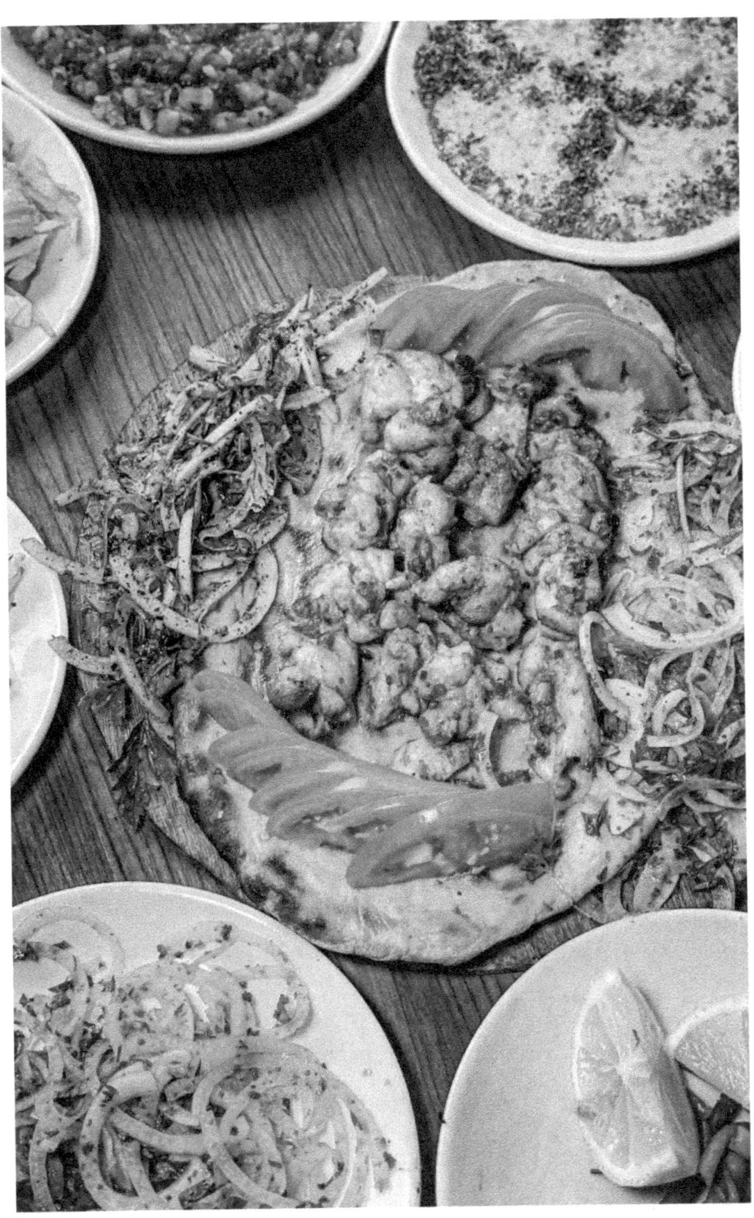

TABLE OF CONTENTS

Chapter 5: Snacks and Appetizers 86

CONCLUSION 142

INTRODUCTION

Our kidneys are the silent powerhouses of our body, diligently filtering waste products and toxins from our blood, keeping us balanced and healthy. But like any hardworking organ, they need the right fuel to function at their best. For individuals with kidney concerns, or those seeking to prevent future issues, a plant-based diet can be a game-changer.

Why Plants are Kidney-Friendly Allies:

- **Lowering the Protein Load:** Animal protein, while essential in moderation, puts extra strain on the kidneys to process waste products like urea. Plant-based proteins, found in legumes, nuts, seeds, and whole grains, are gentler on the kidneys and provide a steady stream of essential amino acids.

- **Keeping Inflammation at Bay**: Chronic inflammation is linked to various health issues, including kidney disease. Plant-based diets are naturally anti-inflammatory, rich in antioxidants and fiber from fruits, vegetables, and whole grains. This helps reduce inflammation throughout the body, including the kidneys.

- **Blood Pressure Balancing Act**: High blood pressure is a major risk factor for kidney disease. Plant-based diets are naturally lower in sodium and saturated fat, while being rich in potassium, magnesium, and fiber – all nutrients known to help regulate blood pressure.

- **Weight Management Matters:** Obesity is another risk factor for kidney disease. Plant-based diets tend to be lower in calorie density and promote satiety, aiding in weight management and reducing the burden on the kidneys.

Building a Kidney-Friendly Vegan Plate:

- **Variety is Key:** Embrace the rainbow! Fill your plate with a diverse range of fruits and vegetables, each offering unique nutrients and antioxidants. Aim for at least five servings per day.

- **Legumes Lead the Way**: Lentils, beans, chickpeas, and tofu are protein powerhouses, packed with fiber and essential minerals. Include them in salads, soups, stews, or as burger patties for a satisfying protein punch.

- **Whole Grains for Steady Energy:** Swap refined grains for quinoa, brown rice, oats, and whole-wheat bread. These complex carbohydrates provide sustained energy and essential nutrients like B vitamins and fiber.

- **Healthy Fats for Flavor and Function:** Nuts, seeds, and avocados are rich in omega-3 fatty acids, which have anti-inflammatory properties. Use them as toppings, dressings, or healthy snacks.

- **Hydration Hero:** Water is essential for optimal kidney function. Aim for eight glasses of water per day, and incorporate hydrating fruits and vegetables like watermelon and cucumber.

Beyond the Plate: Lifestyle Tweaks for Kidney Health:

- **Limit Salt and Processed Foods:** These are often high in sodium and unhealthy fats, both of which can burden the kidneys. Opt for fresh, home-cooked meals and read labels carefully.
- **Get Moving:** Regular physical activity helps regulate blood pressure and overall health, benefiting your kidneys as well. Aim for at least 30 minutes of moderate-intensity exercise most days of the week.
- **Manage Stress:** Chronic stress can contribute to inflammation and other health issues. Practice stress-management techniques like yoga, meditation, or spending time in nature.

By embracing a plant-based lifestyle, rich in colorful fruits, vegetables, whole grains, and legumes, you can nourish your body, protect your kidneys, and cultivate vibrant health from the ground up. So, let's raise a glass of plant-based milk to our hardworking kidneys and embrace the power of plant-based nutrition for a lifetime of well-being!

Chapter 1: 30 Day Meal Plan

Week 1:

Day 1:

- Breakfast: Quinoa Breakfast Bowl
- Lunch: Lentil and Vegetable Stew
- Dinner: Mushroom and Lentil Shepherd's Pie
- Snacks: Roasted Red Pepper Hummus with Veggie Sticks
- Dessert: Vegan Chocolate Avocado Mousse

Day 2:

- Breakfast: Sweet Potato and Spinach Breakfast Hash
- Lunch: Chickpea and Spinach Salad
- Dinner: Vegan Spinach and Artichoke Stuffed Peppers
- Snacks: Vegan Guacamole with Baked Tortilla Chips
- Dessert: Berry and Almond Tart

Day 3:

- Breakfast: Chia Seed Pudding with Berries
- Lunch: Quinoa and Black Bean Bowl
- Dinner: Quinoa and Sweet Potato Chili
- Snacks: Spicy Edamame
- Dessert: Vegan Pumpkin Pie

Day 4:

- Breakfast: Vegan Tofu Scramble
- Lunch: Vegan Caesar Salad with Tempeh
- Dinner: Vegan Eggplant and Zucchini Lasagna
- Snacks: Cucumber and Tomato Salsa
- Dessert: Coconut and Mango Sorbet

Day 5:

- Breakfast: Buckwheat Pancakes with Blueberry Compote
- Lunch: Roasted Vegetable Wrap
- Dinner: Thai Green Curry with Tofu
- Snacks: Vegan Spinach and Artichoke Dip
- Dessert: Vegan Lemon Blueberry Cheesecake

Day 6:

- Breakfast: Avocado and Tomato Toast
- Lunch: Kidney Bean and Kale Soup
- Dinner: Spaghetti Squash with Vegan Bolognese
- Snacks: Crispy Chickpeas with Smoky Paprika
- Dessert: Chocolate-Dipped Strawberries

Day 7:

- Breakfast: Kidney Bean Breakfast Burrito
- Lunch: Brown Rice and Mixed Vegetable Stir-Fry
- Dinner: Stuffed Acorn Squash with Wild Rice
- Snacks: Stuffed Grape Leaves with Quinoa
- Dessert: Vegan Banana Bread Pudding

Week 2:

Day 8:

- Breakfast: Oatmeal with Almond Butter and Banana
- Lunch: Vegan Caprese Salad
- Dinner: Vegan Teriyaki Tempeh Stir-Fry
- Snacks: Vegan Caprese Skewers
- Dessert: Almond and Raspberry Thumbprint Cookies

Day 9:

- Breakfast: Vegan Breakfast Tacos
- Lunch: Sweet Potato and Lentil Curry
- Dinner: Chickpea and Vegetable Tagine
- Snacks: Sweet Potato Fries with Garlic Aioli
- Dessert: Vegan Apple Crisp

Day 10:

- Breakfast: Spinach and Mushroom Vegan Frittata
- Lunch: Mediterranean Chickpea Salad
- Dinner: Vegan Butternut Squash Risotto
- Snacks: Vegan Buffalo Cauliflower Bites
- Dessert: Avocado Lime Vegan Cheesecake Bars

Day 11:

- Breakfast: Millet Porridge with Mixed Berries
- Lunch: Vegan Minestrone Soup
- Dinner: Black Bean and Corn Quesadillas
- Snacks: Avocado and Black Bean Salsa
- Dessert: Chocolate Peanut Butter Energy Bites

Day 12:

- Breakfast: Vegan Banana Nut Muffins
- Lunch: Cauliflower and Chickpea Tacos
- Dinner: Cauliflower Steak with Chimichurri Sauce
- Snacks: Vegan Pesto and Tomato Bruschetta
- Dessert: Vegan Carrot Cake with Cashew Cream Frosting

Day 13:

- Breakfast: Zucchini and Tomato Breakfast Casserole
- Lunch: Spinach and Avocado Salad with Citrus Dressing
- Dinner: Vegan Paella with Mixed Vegetables
- Snacks: Green Pea and Mint Hummus
- Dessert: Blueberry Coconut Bliss Balls

Day 14:

- Breakfast: Almond and Berry Smoothie Bowl
- Lunch: Vegan Eggplant Parmesan
- Dinner: Lentil and Mushroom Stuffed Bell Peppers
- Snacks: Vegan Spring Rolls with Peanut Dipping Sauce

- Dessert: Vegan Peach Cobbler

Week 3:

Day 15:

- Breakfast: Vegan Breakfast Wrap with Hummus
- Lunch: Barley and Vegetable Buddha Bowl
- Dinner: Vegan Sweet Potato Gnocchi
- Snacks: Zucchini and Carrot Fritters
- Dessert: Dark Chocolate Avocado Truffles

Day 16:

- Breakfast: Quinoa Breakfast Bowl
- Lunch: Lentil and Vegetable Stew
- Dinner: Mushroom and Lentil Shepherd's Pie
- Snacks: Roasted Red Pepper Hummus with Veggie Sticks
- Dessert: Vegan Chocolate Avocado Mousse

Day 17:

- Breakfast: Sweet Potato and Spinach Breakfast Hash
- Lunch: Chickpea and Spinach Salad

- Dinner: Vegan Spinach and Artichoke Stuffed Peppers
- Snacks: Vegan Guacamole with Baked Tortilla Chips
- Dessert: Berry and Almond Tart

Day 18:

- Breakfast: Chia Seed Pudding with Berries
- Lunch: Quinoa and Black Bean Bowl
- Dinner: Quinoa and Sweet Potato Chili
- Snacks: Spicy Edamame
- Dessert: Vegan Pumpkin Pie

Day 19:

- Breakfast: Vegan Tofu Scramble
- Lunch: Vegan Caesar Salad with Tempeh
- Dinner: Vegan Eggplant and Zucchini Lasagna
- Snacks: Cucumber and Tomato Salsa
- Dessert: Coconut and Mango Sorbet

Day 20:

- Breakfast: Buckwheat Pancakes with Blueberry Compote
- Lunch: Roasted Vegetable Wrap
- Dinner: Thai Green Curry with Tofu
- Snacks: Vegan Spinach and Artichoke Dip
- Dessert: Vegan Lemon Blueberry Cheesecake

Day 21:

- Breakfast: Avocado and Tomato Toast
- Lunch: Kidney Bean and Kale Soup
- Dinner: Spaghetti Squash with Vegan Bolognese
- Snacks: Crispy Chickpeas with Smoky Paprika
- Dessert: Chocolate-Dipped Strawberries

Week 4:

Day 22:

- Breakfast: Kidney Bean Breakfast Burrito
- Lunch: Brown Rice and Mixed Vegetable Stir-Fry
- Dinner: Stuffed Acorn Squash with Wild Rice
- Snacks: Stuffed Grape Leaves with Quinoa
- Dessert: Vegan Banana Bread Pudding

Day 23:

- Breakfast: Oatmeal with Almond Butter and Banana
- Lunch: Vegan Caprese Salad
- Dinner: Vegan Teriyaki Tempeh Stir-Fry
- Snacks: Vegan Caprese Skewers
- Dessert: Almond and Raspberry Thumbprint Cookies

Day 24:

- Breakfast: Vegan Breakfast Tacos
- Lunch: Sweet Potato and Lentil Curry
- Dinner: Chickpea and Vegetable Tagine
- Snacks: Sweet Potato Fries with Garlic Aioli
- Dessert: Vegan Apple Crisp

Day 25:

- Breakfast: Spinach and Mushroom Vegan Frittata
- Lunch: Mediterranean Chickpea Salad
- Dinner: Vegan Butternut Squash Risotto
- Snacks: Vegan Buffalo Cauliflower Bites
- Dessert: Avocado Lime Vegan Cheesecake Bars

Day 26:

- Breakfast: Millet Porridge with Mixed Berries
- Lunch: Vegan Minestrone Soup
- Dinner: Black Bean and Corn Quesadillas
- Snacks: Avocado and Black Bean Salsa
- Dessert: Chocolate Peanut Butter Energy Bites

Day 27:

- Breakfast: Vegan Banana Nut Muffins
- Lunch: Cauliflower and Chickpea Tacos
- Dinner: Cauliflower Steak with Chimichurri Sauce
- Snacks: Vegan Pesto and Tomato Bruschetta
- Dessert: Vegan Carrot Cake with Cashew Cream Frosting

Day 28:

- Breakfast: Zucchini and Tomato Breakfast Casserole
- Lunch: Spinach and Avocado Salad with Citrus Dressing
- Dinner: Vegan Paella with Mixed Vegetables
- Snacks: Green Pea and Mint Hummus
- Dessert: Blueberry Coconut Bliss Balls

Day 29:

- Breakfast: Almond and Berry Smoothie Bowl
- Lunch: Vegan Eggplant Parmesan
- Dinner: Lentil and Mushroom Stuffed Bell Peppers
- Snacks: Vegan Spring Rolls with Peanut Dipping Sauce
- Dessert: Vegan Peach Cobbler

Day 30:

- Breakfast: Vegan Breakfast Wrap with Hummus
- Lunch: Barley and Vegetable Buddha Bowl
- Dinner: Vegan Sweet Potato Gnocchi
- Snacks: Zucchini and Carrot Fritters
- Dessert: Dark Chocolate Avocado Truffles

Chapter 2: Breakfast Recipes

In this chapter, we've curated a collection of delicious breakfast recipes that not only cater to your taste buds but also align with kidney-friendly dietary guidelines. Each recipe is crafted with care, providing you with a burst of flavors and essential nutrients.

Quinoa Breakfast Bowl

Ingredients:

- 1 cup cooked quinoa
- 1/2 cup diced mango
- 1/4 cup pomegranate seeds
- 2 tablespoons chopped almonds
- 1 teaspoon agave syrup

Instructions:

1. In a bowl, combine cooked quinoa, diced mango, pomegranate seeds, and chopped almonds.
2. Drizzle agave syrup over the mixture and toss gently.
3. Enjoy the refreshing Quinoa Breakfast Bowl!

Nutrition Information:

- Calories: 300
- Protein: 8g
- Carbohydrates: 55g
- Fat: 6g
- Sodium: 10mg
- Potassium: 380mg
- Phosphorus: 150mg
- Portion Size: 1 serving

Sweet Potato and Spinach Breakfast Hash

Ingredients:

- 1 large sweet potato, diced
- 1 cup fresh spinach
- 1/2 red onion, diced
- 1 tablespoon olive oil
- 1/2 teaspoon smoked paprika

Instructions:

1. Heat olive oil in a pan and sauté diced sweet potato until golden brown.

2. Add diced red onion and continue cooking until softened.

3. Stir in fresh spinach and smoked paprika, cooking until spinach wilts.

4. Serve this flavorful Sweet Potato and Spinach Breakfast Hash!

Nutrition Information:

- Calories: 250
- Protein: 5g
- Carbohydrates: 40g
- Fat: 8g
- Sodium: 20mg
- Potassium: 520mg
- Phosphorus: 120mg
- Portion Size: 1 serving

Chia Seed Pudding with Berries

Ingredients:

- 3 tablespoons chia seeds
- 1 cup almond milk
- 1/2 cup mixed berries (strawberries, blueberries, raspberries)
- 1 tablespoon maple syrup

Instructions:

1. Mix chia seeds and almond milk in a bowl, refrigerate overnight.
2. In the morning, layer chia pudding with mixed berries.
3. Drizzle with maple syrup and savor the Chia Seed Pudding with Berries!

Nutrition Information:

- Calories: 180
- Protein: 5g
- Carbohydrates: 25g
- Fat: 8g
- Sodium: 80mg

- Potassium: 160mg
- Phosphorus: 100mg
- Portion Size: 1 serving

Vegan Tofu Scramble

Ingredients:

- 1/2 block firm tofu, crumbled
- 1 cup cherry tomatoes, halved
- 1/4 cup chopped kale
- 1 clove garlic, minced
- 1 tablespoon nutritional yeast

Instructions:

1. Sauté crumbled tofu in a pan until lightly browned.
2. Add cherry tomatoes, chopped kale, minced garlic, and nutritional yeast.
3. Cook until vegetables are tender, creating a delicious Vegan Tofu Scramble!

Nutrition Information:

- Calories: 220
- Protein: 15g

- Carbohydrates: 10g
- Fat: 14g
- Sodium: 30mg
- Potassium: 380mg
- Phosphorus: 200mg
- Portion Size: 1 serving

Buckwheat Pancakes with Blueberry Compote

Ingredients:

- 1 cup buckwheat flour
- 1 tablespoon ground flaxseed
- 1 teaspoon baking powder
- 1 cup almond milk
- 1/2 cup blueberries (for compote)

Instructions:

1. Mix buckwheat flour, ground flaxseed, baking powder, and almond milk in a bowl.
2. Pour batter onto a hot griddle, flipping when bubbles form.

3. Serve with a blueberry compote for delightful Buckwheat Pancakes!

Nutrition Information:

- Calories: 280
- Protein: 8g
- Carbohydrates: 45g
- Fat: 7g
- Sodium: 180mg
- Potassium: 240mg
- Phosphorus: 120mg
- Portion Size: 2 pancakes with compote

Avocado and Tomato Toast

Ingredients:

- 2 slices whole-grain bread
- 1 ripe avocado, mashed
- 1 medium tomato, sliced
- Pinch of salt and pepper
- Sprinkle of nutritional yeast

Instructions:

1. Toast whole-grain bread slices until golden brown.

2. Spread mashed avocado on the toast, top with tomato slices.

3. Season with salt, pepper, and a sprinkle of nutritional yeast.

4. Enjoy the simplicity of Avocado and Tomato Toast!

Nutrition Information:

- Calories: 220
- Protein: 7g
- Carbohydrates: 30g
- Fat: 10g
- Sodium: 180mg
- Potassium: 480mg
- Phosphorus: 150mg
- Portion Size: 1 serving

Kidney Bean Breakfast Burrito

Ingredients:

- 1 cup cooked kidney beans
- 1 whole-grain tortilla

- 1/4 cup diced bell peppers
- 2 tablespoons salsa
- 1/4 cup chopped cilantro

Instructions:

1. Warm kidney beans and whole-grain tortilla.
2. Fill tortilla with kidney beans, diced bell peppers, salsa, and cilantro.
3. Roll into a burrito and relish the Kidney Bean Breakfast Burrito!

Nutrition Information:

- Calories: 300
- Protein: 12g
- Carbohydrates: 50g
- Fat: 6g
- Sodium: 320mg
- Potassium: 380mg
- Phosphorus: 140mg
- Portion Size: 1 burrito

Oatmeal with Almond Butter and Banana

Ingredients:

- 1/2 cup rolled oats
- 1 cup almond milk
- 1 tablespoon almond butter
- 1 ripe banana, sliced
- Drizzle of maple syrup

Instructions:

1. Cook rolled oats in almond milk until creamy.
2. Top with almond butter, sliced banana, and a drizzle of maple syrup.
3. Delight in the heartiness of Oatmeal with Almond Butter and Banana!

Nutrition Information:

- Calories: 280
- Protein: 8g
- Carbohydrates: 45g
- Fat: 10g
- Sodium: 80mg

- Potassium: 380mg
- Phosphorus: 180mg
- Portion Size: 1 serving

Vegan Breakfast Tacos

Ingredients:

- 3 corn tortillas
- 1/2 cup black beans, cooked
- 1/4 cup diced tomatoes
- 2 tablespoons guacamole
- Fresh cilantro for garnish

Instructions:

1. Warm corn tortillas and black beans.
2. Fill tortillas with black beans, diced tomatoes, and guacamole.
3. Garnish with fresh cilantro and enjoy the Vegan Breakfast Tacos!

Nutrition Information:

- Calories: 250
- Protein: 10g

- Carbohydrates: 35g
- Fat: 8g
- Sodium: 180mg
- Potassium: 380mg
- Phosphorus: 160mg
- Portion Size: 3 tacos

Spinach and Mushroom Vegan Frittata

Ingredients:

- 1 cup chickpea flour
- 1 1/2 cups water
- 1 cup fresh spinach, chopped
- 1/2 cup mushrooms, sliced
- 1/4 cup nutritional yeast

Instructions:

1. Whisk chickpea flour and water to make a batter.
2. Mix in chopped spinach, sliced mushrooms, and nutritional yeast.
3. Pour into a greased baking dish and bake until set.

4. Slice and serve the savory Spinach and Mushroom Vegan Frittata!

Nutrition Information:

- Calories: 220
- Protein: 15g
- Carbohydrates: 25g
- Fat: 8g
- Sodium: 180mg
- Potassium: 380mg
- Phosphorus: 160mg
- Portion Size: 1 serving

Millet Porridge with Mixed Berries

Ingredients:

- 1/2 cup millet, rinsed
- 2 cups almond milk
- 1 cup mixed berries (strawberries, blueberries, raspberries)
- 1 tablespoon agave syrup

Instructions:

1. Cook millet in almond milk until soft and creamy.

2. Top with mixed berries and drizzle with agave syrup.

3. Enjoy the warmth of Millet Porridge with Mixed Berries!

Nutrition Information:

- Calories: 230

- Protein: 5g

- Carbohydrates: 45g

- Fat: 4g

- Sodium: 70mg

- Potassium: 240mg

- Phosphorus: 120mg

- Portion Size: 1 serving

Vegan Banana Nut Muffins

Ingredients:

- 1 1/2 cups whole wheat flour

- 1 teaspoon baking powder

- 1/2 teaspoon baking soda

- 1/2 cup mashed ripe bananas

- 1/4 cup chopped walnuts

Instructions:

1. Mix whole wheat flour, baking powder, and baking soda in a bowl.
2. Add mashed bananas and chopped walnuts, stir until just combined.
3. Spoon into muffin cups and bake until golden brown.
4. Relish the goodness of Vegan Banana Nut Muffins!

Nutrition Information:

- Calories: 180
- Protein: 5g
- Carbohydrates: 30g
- Fat: 6g
- Sodium: 160mg
- Potassium: 240mg
- Phosphorus: 100mg
- Portion Size: 1 muffin

Zucchini and Tomato Breakfast Casserole

Ingredients:

- 2 zucchinis, sliced
- 1 cup cherry tomatoes, halved
- 1 cup spinach, chopped
- 1 cup chickpea flour
- 1 1/2 cups almond milk

Instructions:

1. Layer zucchini slices, cherry tomatoes, and chopped spinach in a baking dish.
2. Whisk chickpea flour and almond milk, pour over the vegetables.
3. Bake until set, creating the Zucchini and Tomato Breakfast Casserole!

Nutrition Information:

- Calories: 240
- Protein: 12g
- Carbohydrates: 30g
- Fat: 10g

- Sodium: 180mg

- Potassium: 480mg

- Phosphorus: 160mg

- Portion Size: 1 serving

Almond and Berry Smoothie Bowl

Ingredients:

- 1 frozen banana

- 1/2 cup mixed berries (strawberries, blueberries, raspberries)

- 1 cup almond milk

- 2 tablespoons almond butter

- Toppings: sliced almonds, chia seeds, fresh berries

Instructions:

1. Blend frozen banana, mixed berries, almond milk, and almond butter.

2. Pour into a bowl and add toppings for a delightful Almond and Berry Smoothie Bowl!

Nutrition Information:

- Calories: 280

- Protein: 8g

- Carbohydrates: 40g

- Fat: 12g

- Sodium: 80mg

- Potassium: 420mg

- Phosphorus: 120mg

- Portion Size: 1 serving

Vegan Breakfast Wrap with Hummus

Ingredients:

- 1 whole-grain tortilla

- 2 tablespoons hummus

- 1/4 cup shredded carrots

- 1/4 cup cucumber, thinly sliced

- Handful of baby spinach

Instructions:

1. Spread hummus on a whole-grain tortilla.

2. Layer with shredded carrots, thinly sliced cucumber, and baby spinach.

3. Roll into a wrap and enjoy the simplicity of the Vegan Breakfast Wrap with Hummus!

Nutrition Information:

- Calories: 220
- Protein: 7g
- Carbohydrates: 30g
- Fat: 8g
- Sodium: 180mg
- Potassium: 380mg
- Phosphorus: 140mg
- Portion Size: 1 wrap

Chapter 3: Lunch Recipes

These recipes are carefully curated to embrace the richness of plant-based ingredients, ensuring a burst of nutritional goodness in every bite. Let's dive into a world of delicious and nourishing vegan lunches.

Lentil and Vegetable Stew

Ingredients:

- 1 cup green lentils, rinsed
- 2 carrots, diced
- 1 onion, chopped
- 3 cloves garlic, minced
- 1 zucchini, sliced
- 1 can (14 oz) diced tomatoes
- 4 cups vegetable broth
- 1 teaspoon cumin
- 1 teaspoon paprika
- Salt and pepper to taste

Instructions:

1. In a large pot, sauté onions and garlic until fragrant.
2. Add carrots, zucchini, lentils, tomatoes, and vegetable broth.
3. Season with cumin, paprika, salt, and pepper.
4. Simmer for 30-40 minutes until lentils are tender.
5. Serve hot and enjoy!

Nutrition Information:

- Calories: 250
- Protein: 15g
- Carbohydrates: 45g
- Fat: 2g
- Sodium: 600mg
- Potassium: 700mg
- Phosphorus: 150mg
- Portion Size: 1 cup

Chickpea and Spinach Salad

Ingredients:

- 2 cups chickpeas, cooked
- 4 cups fresh spinach

- 1 cucumber, sliced
- 1 cup cherry tomatoes, halved
- 1/4 cup red onion, thinly sliced
- 1/3 cup balsamic vinaigrette dressing

Instructions:

1. In a large bowl, combine chickpeas, spinach, cucumber, tomatoes, and red onion.
2. Drizzle with balsamic vinaigrette dressing and toss gently.
3. Chill for 15 minutes before serving.

Nutrition Information:

- Calories: 280
- Protein: 12g
- Carbohydrates: 40g
- Fat: 8g
- Sodium: 450mg
- Potassium: 600mg
- Phosphorus: 120mg
- Portion Size: 2 cups

Quinoa and Black Bean Bowl

Ingredients:

- 1 cup quinoa, cooked
- 1 can (15 oz) black beans, drained and rinsed
- 1 cup corn kernels
- 1 red bell pepper, diced
- 1/4 cup cilantro, chopped
- 1 lime, juiced
- Salt and cumin to taste

Instructions:

1. In a bowl, combine quinoa, black beans, corn, and red bell pepper.
2. Add cilantro, lime juice, salt, and cumin. Mix well.
3. Serve at room temperature or chilled.

Nutrition Information:

- Calories: 320
- Protein: 15g
- Carbohydrates: 60g
- Fat: 4g
- Sodium: 300mg

- Potassium: 550mg
- Phosphorus: 200mg
- Portion Size: 1.5 cups

Vegan Caesar Salad with Tempeh

Ingredients:

- 1 head romaine lettuce, chopped
- 1 cup cherry tomatoes, halved
- 1/2 cup croutons (whole wheat)
- 1/3 cup vegan Caesar dressing
- 1 cup tempeh, cubed and sautéed

Instructions:

1. In a large bowl, combine romaine lettuce, cherry tomatoes, and croutons.
2. Toss with vegan Caesar dressing until well coated.
3. Top with sautéed tempeh cubes.
4. Serve immediately for a crisp delight.

Nutrition Information:

- Calories: 280
- Protein: 14g

- Carbohydrates: 30g

- Fat: 14g

- Sodium: 450mg

- Potassium: 400mg

- Phosphorus: 180mg

- Portion Size: 2 cups

Roasted Vegetable Wrap

Ingredients:

- 1 whole-grain tortilla

- 1/2 cup hummus

- 1 cup mixed roasted vegetables (zucchini, bell peppers, eggplant)

- Handful of fresh spinach

- 1 tablespoon tahini

Instructions:

1. Spread hummus on the tortilla.

2. Add roasted vegetables and fresh spinach.

3. Drizzle with tahini.

4. Roll tightly into a wrap.

5. Slice in half and enjoy!

Nutrition Information:

- Calories: 320
- Protein: 10g
- Carbohydrates: 45g
- Fat: 12g
- Sodium: 380mg
- Potassium: 450mg
- Phosphorus: 160mg
- Portion Size: 1 wrap

Kidney Bean and Kale Soup

Ingredients:

- 2 cups kidney beans, cooked
- 4 cups kale, chopped
- 1 onion, diced
- 3 cloves garlic, minced
- 1 carrot, sliced
- 1 can (14 oz) crushed tomatoes
- 6 cups vegetable broth
- 1 teaspoon Italian seasoning
- Salt and pepper to taste

Instructions:

1. In a large pot, sauté onions and garlic until softened.
2. Add kale, kidney beans, carrot, tomatoes, and vegetable broth.
3. Season with Italian seasoning, salt, and pepper.
4. Simmer for 25-30 minutes.
5. Ladle into bowls and serve hot.

Nutrition Information:

- Calories: 270
- Protein: 13g
- Carbohydrates: 50g
- Fat: 1g
- Sodium: 580mg
- Potassium: 700mg
- Phosphorus: 200mg
- Portion Size: 1.5 cups

Brown Rice and Mixed Vegetable Stir-Fry

Ingredients:

- 1 cup brown rice, cooked
- 1 cup broccoli florets
- 1 bell pepper, sliced
- 1 carrot, julienned
- 1 cup snap peas
- 2 tablespoons soy sauce (low sodium)
- 1 tablespoon sesame oil
- 1 teaspoon ginger, minced

Instructions:

1. In a wok or large pan, heat sesame oil.
2. Stir-fry broccoli, bell pepper, carrot, and snap peas until crisp-tender.
3. Add cooked brown rice and ginger, stir well.
4. Pour soy sauce over the mixture and toss until evenly coated.
5. Serve hot and savor the flavors.

Nutrition Information:

- Calories: 290
- Protein: 8g
- Carbohydrates: 55g
- Fat: 6g
- Sodium: 550mg
- Potassium: 450mg
- Phosphorus: 140mg
- Portion Size: 1.5 cups

Vegan Caprese Salad

Ingredients:

- 4 large tomatoes, sliced
- 1 cup vegan mozzarella, sliced
- Fresh basil leaves
- Balsamic glaze
- Salt and pepper to taste

Instructions:

1. Arrange tomato and mozzarella slices on a plate.
2. Tuck fresh basil leaves between slices.
3. Drizzle with balsamic glaze.

4. Season with salt and pepper.

5. Serve as a refreshing salad.

Nutrition Information:

- Calories: 220
- Protein: 6g
- Carbohydrates: 10g
- Fat: 16g
- Sodium: 400mg
- Potassium: 450mg
- Phosphorus: 120mg
- Portion Size: 1 cup

Sweet Potato and Lentil Curry

Ingredients:

- 2 cups sweet potatoes, cubed
- 1 cup red lentils, rinsed
- 1 onion, diced
- 3 cloves garlic, minced
- 1 can (14 oz) coconut milk
- 2 tablespoons curry powder
- 1 teaspoon turmeric

- Salt and pepper to taste

Instructions:

1. In a pot, sauté onions and garlic until golden.
2. Add sweet potatoes, lentils, coconut milk, and spices.
3. Simmer for 20-25 minutes until sweet potatoes are tender.
4. Season with salt and pepper.
5. Serve over rice and enjoy!

Nutrition Information:

- Calories: 330
- Protein: 15g
- Carbohydrates: 50g
- Fat: 8g
- Sodium: 380mg
- Potassium: 700mg
- Phosphorus: 180mg
- Portion Size: 1.5 cups

Mediterranean Chickpea Salad

Ingredients:

- 2 cans (15 oz each) chickpeas, drained and rinsed
- 1 cucumber, diced
- 1 cup cherry tomatoes, halved
- 1/2 red onion, finely chopped
- 1/2 cup Kalamata olives, sliced
- 1/3 cup fresh parsley, chopped
- 1/4 cup extra virgin olive oil
- 2 tablespoons red wine vinegar
- Salt and pepper to taste

Instructions:

1. In a large bowl, combine chickpeas, cucumber, tomatoes, red onion, olives, and parsley.
2. In a small bowl, whisk together olive oil, red wine vinegar, salt, and pepper.
3. Pour the dressing over the salad and toss gently.
4. Chill before serving for enhanced flavors.

Nutrition Information:

- Calories: 280

- Protein: 10g

- Carbohydrates: 30g

- Fat: 14g

- Sodium: 500mg

- Potassium: 450mg

- Phosphorus: 140mg

- Portion Size: 1.5 cups

Vegan Minestrone Soup

Ingredients:

- 1 cup whole wheat pasta, cooked

- 1 can (15 oz) kidney beans, drained and rinsed

- 1 cup zucchini, diced

- 1 cup carrots, sliced

- 1 cup celery, chopped

- 1 can (14 oz) diced tomatoes

- 6 cups vegetable broth

- 1 teaspoon dried oregano

- 1 teaspoon dried basil

- Salt and pepper to taste

Instructions:

1. In a pot, combine pasta, kidney beans, zucchini, carrots, celery, tomatoes, and vegetable broth.
2. Season with oregano, basil, salt, and pepper.
3. Simmer for 15-20 minutes until vegetables are tender.
4. Serve hot and enjoy this hearty minestrone.

Nutrition Information:

- Calories: 320
- Protein: 15g
- Carbohydrates: 60g
- Fat: 2g
- Sodium: 580mg
- Potassium: 700mg
- Phosphorus: 150mg
- Portion Size: 1.5 cups

Cauliflower and Chickpea Tacos

Ingredients:

- 2 cups cauliflower florets
- 1 can (15 oz) chickpeas, drained and rinsed

- 1 tablespoon olive oil
- 1 teaspoon chili powder
- 1/2 teaspoon cumin
- 1/2 teaspoon smoked paprika
- 1/4 teaspoon garlic powder
- Corn tortillas
- Toppings: shredded lettuce, salsa, avocado

Instructions:

1. Toss cauliflower and chickpeas with olive oil and spices.
2. Roast in the oven at 400°F (200°C) for 20 minutes.
3. Fill corn tortillas with the roasted mixture.
4. Top with shredded lettuce, salsa, and avocado.
5. Enjoy these flavorful and crunchy tacos!

Nutrition Information:

- Calories: 280
- Protein: 10g
- Carbohydrates: 40g
- Fat: 10g
- Sodium: 450mg

- Potassium: 500mg
- Phosphorus: 140mg
- Portion Size: 2 tacos

Spinach and Avocado Salad with Citrus Dressing

Ingredients:

- 4 cups fresh spinach
- 1 avocado, sliced
- 1 cup cherry tomatoes, halved
- 1/4 cup red onion, thinly sliced
- 1/3 cup walnuts, chopped
- Dressing: 2 tablespoons orange juice, 1 tablespoon lemon juice, 2 tablespoons olive oil, salt, and pepper

Instructions:

1. In a large bowl, combine spinach, avocado, tomatoes, red onion, and walnuts.
2. In a small bowl, whisk together orange juice, lemon juice, olive oil, salt, and pepper.

3. Drizzle the citrus dressing over the salad and toss gently.

4. Serve immediately for a refreshing burst of flavors.

Nutrition Information:

- Calories: 290
- Protein: 6g
- Carbohydrates: 20g
- Fat: 22g
- Sodium: 120mg
- Potassium: 600mg
- Phosphorus: 130mg
- Portion Size: 2 cups

Vegan Eggplant Parmesan

Ingredients:

- 2 large eggplants, sliced
- 1 cup whole wheat breadcrumbs
- 1 cup marinara sauce
- 1 cup vegan mozzarella, shredded
- 1/4 cup nutritional yeast
- Fresh basil for garnish

Instructions:

1. Preheat the oven to 375°F (190°C).
2. Dip eggplant slices in breadcrumbs and arrange in a baking dish.
3. Top with marinara sauce, vegan mozzarella, and nutritional yeast.
4. Bake for 25-30 minutes until golden and bubbly.
5. Garnish with fresh basil before serving.

Nutrition Information:

- Calories: 250
- Protein: 8g
- Carbohydrates: 40g
- Fat: 8g
- Sodium: 450mg
- Potassium: 550mg
- Phosphorus: 180mg
- Portion Size: 1 cup

Barley and Vegetable Buddha Bowl

Ingredients:

- 1 cup cooked barley

- 1 cup roasted sweet potatoes
- 1 cup steamed broccoli florets
- 1/2 cup shredded carrots
- 1/4 cup tahini dressing
- Sprinkle of sesame seeds

Instructions:

1. Arrange cooked barley, roasted sweet potatoes, broccoli, and shredded carrots in a bowl.
2. Drizzle with tahini dressing.
3. Sprinkle sesame seeds on top for added crunch.
4. Dive into this wholesome Buddha bowl!

Nutrition Information:

- Calories: 310
- Protein: 9g
- Carbohydrates: 50g
- Fat: 10g
- Sodium: 180mg
- Potassium: 600mg
- Phosphorus: 160mg
- Portion Size: 1.5 cups

Chapter 4: Dinner Recipes

Here, we will explore a delightful array of plant-based wonders that not only tantalize the taste buds but also cater to kidney-friendly nutritional needs. Each dish is crafted with precision, balancing flavors, textures, and the essential nutrients your body craves.

Mushroom and Lentil Shepherd's Pie

Ingredients:

- 1 cup lentils, rinsed
- 2 cups mushrooms, diced
- 1 onion, finely chopped
- 2 carrots, peeled and diced
- 3 cloves garlic, minced
- 1 cup frozen peas
- 4 cups mashed sweet potatoes
- 1 tablespoon olive oil
- 1 teaspoon thyme
- Salt and pepper to taste

Instructions:

1. Preheat oven to 375°F (190°C).
2. Cook lentils according to package instructions.
3. In a pan, sauté mushrooms, onions, carrots, and garlic in olive oil until tender.
4. Mix in cooked lentils, peas, thyme, salt, and pepper.
5. Transfer the mixture to a baking dish and top with mashed sweet potatoes.
6. Bake for 25-30 minutes or until the top is golden brown.

Nutrition Information (per serving):

- Calories: 350
- Protein: 15g
- Carbohydrates: 65g
- Fat: 5g
- Sodium: 300mg
- Potassium: 800mg
- Phosphorus: 150mg
- Portion size: 1 cup

Vegan Spinach and Artichoke Stuffed Peppers

Ingredients:

- 4 large bell peppers, halved
- 2 cups fresh spinach, chopped
- 1 can artichoke hearts, drained and chopped
- 1 cup cooked quinoa
- 1 cup vegan cream cheese
- 1/2 cup nutritional yeast
- 2 cloves garlic, minced
- Salt and pepper to taste

Instructions:

1. Preheat oven to 375°F (190°C).
2. Boil bell peppers for 5 minutes, then drain.
3. In a bowl, combine spinach, artichokes, quinoa, cream cheese, nutritional yeast, garlic, salt, and pepper.
4. Stuff each pepper half with the mixture.
5. Bake for 20-25 minutes or until peppers are tender.

Nutrition Information (per serving):

- Calories: 250
- Protein: 10g
- Carbohydrates: 30g
- Fat: 12g
- Sodium: 400mg
- Potassium: 600mg
- Phosphorus: 120mg
- Portion size: 2 halves

Quinoa and Sweet Potato Chili

Ingredients:

- 1 cup quinoa, rinsed
- 2 sweet potatoes, diced
- 1 can black beans, drained and rinsed
- 1 can diced tomatoes
- 1 onion, chopped
- 3 cloves garlic, minced
- 1 tablespoon chili powder
- 1 teaspoon cumin
- Salt and pepper to taste

Instructions:

1. Cook quinoa according to package instructions.

2. In a large pot, sauté onions and garlic until fragrant.

3. Add sweet potatoes, black beans, diced tomatoes, chili powder, cumin, salt, and pepper.

4. Simmer until sweet potatoes are tender.

5. Stir in cooked quinoa and let it simmer for an additional 10 minutes.

Nutrition Information (per serving):

- Calories: 320
- Protein: 12g
- Carbohydrates: 60g
- Fat: 3g
- Sodium: 500mg
- Potassium: 700mg
- Phosphorus: 200mg
- Portion size: 1 cup

Vegan Eggplant and Zucchini Lasagna

Ingredients:

- 2 medium eggplants, thinly sliced
- 2 zucchinis, thinly sliced
- 2 cups tomato sauce
- 1 cup vegan ricotta cheese
- 1 cup vegan mozzarella, shredded
- 2 tablespoons olive oil
- 2 teaspoons dried oregano
- Salt and pepper to taste

Instructions:

1. Preheat oven to 375°F (190°C).
2. In a baking dish, layer eggplant and zucchini slices.
3. Spread a layer of tomato sauce, followed by dollops of vegan ricotta and a sprinkle of vegan mozzarella.
4. Repeat the layers until ingredients are used, ending with a layer of tomato sauce and mozzarella.
5. Drizzle olive oil, sprinkle oregano, salt, and pepper on top.
6. Bake for 30-35 minutes or until bubbly and golden.

Nutrition Information (per serving):

- Calories: 280

- Protein: 8g

- Carbohydrates: 30g

- Fat: 15g

- Sodium: 450mg

- Potassium: 600mg

- Phosphorus: 120mg

- Portion size: 1 slice

Thai Green Curry with Tofu

Ingredients:

- 1 block extra-firm tofu, cubed

- 1 can coconut milk

- 2 tablespoons green curry paste

- 1 cup broccoli florets

- 1 red bell pepper, sliced

- 1 cup snap peas

- 1 tablespoon soy sauce

- 1 tablespoon maple syrup

- Fresh basil leaves for garnish

Instructions:

1. Press tofu to remove excess water and cube.

2. In a pan, combine coconut milk and green curry paste. Bring to a simmer.

3. Add tofu, broccoli, bell pepper, snap peas, soy sauce, and maple syrup.

4. Simmer until vegetables are tender and tofu is heated through.

5. Garnish with fresh basil before serving.

Nutrition Information (per serving):

- Calories: 320

- Protein: 15g

- Carbohydrates: 20g

- Fat: 20g

- Sodium: 400mg

- Potassium: 550mg

- Phosphorus: 180mg

- Portion size: 1 cup

Spaghetti Squash with Vegan Bolognese

Ingredients:

- 1 large spaghetti squash, halved
- 2 cups vegan bolognese sauce
- 1 tablespoon olive oil
- 1 onion, finely chopped
- 2 carrots, grated
- 2 celery stalks, diced
- 2 cloves garlic, minced
- 1 can lentils, drained and rinsed
- 1 can crushed tomatoes
- 1 teaspoon dried basil
- Salt and pepper to taste

Instructions:

1. Preheat oven to 375°F (190°C).
2. Roast spaghetti squash halves for 40-45 minutes.
3. In a pan, sauté onions, carrots, celery, and garlic in olive oil.
4. Add lentils, crushed tomatoes, basil, salt, and pepper. Simmer until flavors meld.

5. Scrape spaghetti squash with a fork to create "noodles" and top with vegan bolognese.

Nutrition Information (per serving):

- Calories: 280
- Protein: 12g
- Carbohydrates: 40g
- Fat: 8g
- Sodium: 450mg
- Potassium: 700mg
- Phosphorus: 160mg
- Portion size: 1 cup

Stuffed Acorn Squash with Wild Rice

Ingredients:

- 3 acorn squashes, halved
- 1 cup wild rice, cooked
- 1 cup kale, chopped
- 1/2 cup dried cranberries
- 1/2 cup pecans, chopped
- 1 tablespoon olive oil
- 1 teaspoon dried sage

- Salt and pepper to taste

Instructions:

1. Preheat oven to 375°F (190°C).
2. Roast acorn squashes for 40-45 minutes.
3. In a pan, sauté kale in olive oil until wilted.
4. Mix cooked wild rice, sautéed kale, dried cranberries, pecans, sage, salt, and pepper.
5. Fill each acorn squash half with the wild rice mixture.

Nutrition Information (per serving):

- Calories: 300
- Protein: 7g
- Carbohydrates: 60g
- Fat: 8g
- Sodium: 200mg
- Potassium: 700mg
- Phosphorus: 140mg
- Portion size: 1 half

Vegan Teriyaki Tempeh Stir-Fry

Ingredients:

- 1 block tempeh, cubed
- 2 cups broccoli florets
- 1 red bell pepper, sliced
- 1 carrot, julienned
- 1 cup snow peas
- 1/4 cup soy sauce
- 2 tablespoons maple syrup
- 1 tablespoon sesame oil
- 2 cloves garlic, minced
- 1 teaspoon ginger, grated
- Sesame seeds for garnish

Instructions:

1. In a pan, sauté tempeh until golden brown.
2. Add broccoli, bell pepper, carrot, and snow peas. Cook until vegetables are tender-crisp.
3. In a bowl, mix soy sauce, maple syrup, sesame oil, garlic, and ginger. Pour over the stir-fry.
4. Toss until well coated and heated through.
5. Garnish with sesame seeds before serving.

Nutrition Information (per serving):

- Calories: 280
- Protein: 15g
- Carbohydrates: 30g
- Fat: 12g
- Sodium: 600mg
- Potassium: 550mg
- Phosphorus: 200mg
- Portion size: 1 cup

Chickpea and Vegetable Tagine

Ingredients:

- 1 can chickpeas, drained and rinsed
- 1 eggplant, diced
- 2 zucchinis, sliced
- 1 bell pepper, chopped
- 1 onion, finely chopped
- 3 cloves garlic, minced
- 1 can diced tomatoes
- 1 cup vegetable broth
- 1 teaspoon ground cumin
- 1 teaspoon ground coriander

- 1/2 teaspoon cinnamon
- Salt and pepper to taste

Instructions:

1. In a tagine or large pot, sauté onions and garlic until softened.
2. Add chickpeas, eggplant, zucchinis, bell pepper, diced tomatoes, vegetable broth, cumin, coriander, cinnamon, salt, and pepper.
3. Simmer for 20-25 minutes or until vegetables are tender.

Nutrition Information (per serving):

- Calories: 320
- Protein: 14g
- Carbohydrates: 55g
- Fat: 5g
- Sodium: 500mg
- Potassium: 800mg
- Phosphorus: 160mg
- Portion size: 1 cup

Vegan Butternut Squash Risotto

Ingredients:

- 1 cup Arborio rice
- 2 cups butternut squash, diced
- 1 onion, finely chopped
- 3 cups vegetable broth
- 1/2 cup dry white wine
- 1/4 cup nutritional yeast
- 2 tablespoons olive oil
- 1 teaspoon thyme
- Salt and pepper to taste

Instructions:

1. In a pan, sauté onions in olive oil until translucent.
2. Add Arborio rice and cook until lightly toasted.
3. Pour in white wine and stir until absorbed.
4. Gradually add vegetable broth, one ladle at a time, stirring frequently.
5. Add butternut squash, nutritional yeast, thyme, salt, and pepper.
6. Continue adding broth and stirring until rice is creamy and cooked.

Nutrition Information (per serving):

- Calories: 300
- Protein: 6g
- Carbohydrates: 60g
- Fat: 5g
- Sodium: 500mg
- Potassium: 600mg
- Phosphorus: 120mg
- Portion size: 1 cup

Black Bean and Corn Quesadillas

Ingredients:

- 1 can black beans, drained and rinsed
- 1 cup corn kernels
- 1 red onion, diced
- 1 bell pepper, diced
- 1 teaspoon cumin
- 1 teaspoon chili powder
- 4 whole wheat tortillas
- 1 cup vegan cheese, shredded
- Fresh cilantro for garnish

Instructions:

1. In a bowl, mix black beans, corn, red onion, bell pepper, cumin, and chili powder.
2. Place a tortilla on a griddle or pan, add a portion of the bean mixture, and sprinkle with vegan cheese.
3. Top with another tortilla and cook until golden brown on both sides.
4. Repeat for remaining quesadillas.
5. Garnish with fresh cilantro before serving.

Nutrition Information (per serving):

- Calories: 280
- Protein: 10g
- Carbohydrates: 45g
- Fat: 8g
- Sodium: 400mg
- Potassium: 550mg
- Phosphorus: 180mg
- Portion size: 1 quesadilla

Cauliflower Steak with Chimichurri Sauce

Ingredients:

- 2 cauliflower heads, sliced into steaks
- 1 cup cherry tomatoes, halved
- 1 cup green beans, blanched
- 1/2 cup fresh parsley, chopped
- 3 cloves garlic, minced
- 1/4 cup red wine vinegar
- 1/2 cup olive oil
- Salt and pepper to taste

Instructions:

1. Brush cauliflower steaks with olive oil and season with salt and pepper.
2. Grill or roast until tender and golden brown.
3. In a bowl, mix cherry tomatoes, green beans, parsley, garlic, red wine vinegar, and olive oil for chimichurri sauce.
4. Serve cauliflower steaks topped with chimichurri.

Nutrition Information (per serving):

- Calories: 250
- Protein: 6g
- Carbohydrates: 25g
- Fat: 15g
- Sodium: 300mg
- Potassium: 700mg
- Phosphorus: 120mg
- Portion size: 1 steak

Vegan Paella with Mixed Vegetables

Ingredients:

- 1 cup Arborio rice
- 1 onion, finely chopped
- 2 cloves garlic, minced
- 1 red bell pepper, sliced
- 1 cup cherry tomatoes, halved
- 1 cup artichoke hearts, quartered
- 1 cup green peas
- 1/2 teaspoon saffron threads
- 1 teaspoon smoked paprika
- 2 cups vegetable broth

- 2 tablespoons olive oil

- Lemon wedges for serving

Instructions:

1. In a paella pan or large skillet, sauté onions and garlic in olive oil until softened.
2. Add Arborio rice and sauté until translucent.
3. Stir in bell pepper, cherry tomatoes, artichoke hearts, green peas, saffron, and smoked paprika.
4. Pour in vegetable broth and bring to a simmer.
5. Cook until rice is tender and the liquid is absorbed.
6. Serve with lemon wedges.

Nutrition Information (per serving):

- Calories: 320

- Protein: 6g

- Carbohydrates: 65g

- Fat: 6g

- Sodium: 600mg

- Potassium: 500mg

- Phosphorus: 100mg

- Portion size: 1 cup

Lentil and Mushroom Stuffed Bell Peppers

Ingredients:

- 4 large bell peppers, halved
- 1 cup green lentils, cooked
- 1 cup mushrooms, finely chopped
- 1 onion, diced
- 2 cloves garlic, minced
- 1 can diced tomatoes
- 1 teaspoon dried oregano
- 1 teaspoon smoked paprika
- Salt and pepper to taste
- 1 cup vegan cheese, shredded

Instructions:

1. Preheat oven to 375°F (190°C).
2. Boil bell peppers for 5 minutes, then drain.
3. In a pan, sauté onions and garlic until fragrant.
4. Add mushrooms, lentils, diced tomatoes, oregano, smoked paprika, salt, and pepper.
5. Stuff each pepper half with the lentil and mushroom mixture.

6. Top with vegan cheese and bake for 20-25 minutes.

Nutrition Information (per serving):

- Calories: 280
- Protein: 14g
- Carbohydrates: 40g
- Fat: 8g
- Sodium: 450mg
- Potassium: 600mg
- Phosphorus: 120mg
- Portion size: 2 halves

Vegan Sweet Potato Gnocchi

Ingredients:

- 2 large sweet potatoes, baked and mashed
- 2 cups all-purpose flour
- 1/2 teaspoon salt
- Vegan butter and sage for serving

Instructions:

1. In a large bowl, combine mashed sweet potatoes, flour, and salt.

2. Knead the mixture until a dough forms.

3. Divide the dough into sections and roll into ropes.

4. Cut the ropes into bite-sized pieces to form gnocchi.

5. Boil the gnocchi until they float to the surface.

6. In a pan, sauté cooked gnocchi in vegan butter and
    sage.

Nutrition Information (per serving):

- Calories: 250
- Protein: 5g
- Carbohydrates: 55g
- Fat: 1g
- Sodium: 300mg
- Potassium: 450mg
- Phosphorus: 90mg
- Portion size: 1 cup

Chapter 5: Snacks and Appetizers

These recipes are not just a feast for the taste buds but are crafted with utmost care for those seeking kidney-friendly vegan delights. Get ready to savor a symphony of flavors as we present unique recipes that redefine snacking while keeping nutritional considerations in mind.

Roasted Red Pepper Hummus with Veggie Sticks

Ingredients:

- 1 can (15 oz) chickpeas, drained and rinsed
- 1 large red bell pepper, roasted and peeled
- 2 cloves garlic, minced
- 3 tablespoons tahini
- 2 tablespoons lemon juice
- 2 tablespoons olive oil
- Salt and pepper to taste
- Assorted veggie sticks for dipping

Instructions:

1. In a food processor, combine chickpeas, roasted red pepper, garlic, tahini, and lemon juice.
2. Blend until smooth, drizzling in olive oil as it processes.
3. Season with salt and pepper to taste.
4. Serve with an assortment of veggie sticks for a refreshing crunch.

Nutrition Information (per serving):

- Calories: 120
- Protein: 4g
- Carbohydrates: 15g
- Fat: 6g
- Sodium: 180mg
- Potassium: 160mg
- Phosphorus: 70mg
- Portion Size: 2 tablespoons hummus with veggies

Vegan Guacamole with Baked Tortilla Chips

Ingredients:

- 3 ripe avocados, mashed
- 1 medium tomato, diced
- 1/4 cup red onion, finely chopped
- 2 cloves garlic, minced
- 1 lime, juiced
- Salt and pepper to taste
- Whole grain tortillas for chips

Instructions:

1. In a bowl, combine mashed avocados, diced tomato, red onion, minced garlic, and lime juice.
2. Mix well and season with salt and pepper to taste.
3. Slice tortillas into triangles, bake until crispy.
4. Serve guacamole with baked tortilla chips.

Nutrition Information (per serving):

- Calories: 150
- Protein: 2g
- Carbohydrates: 12g

- Fat: 11g

- Sodium: 80mg

- Potassium: 370mg

- Phosphorus: 50mg

- Portion Size: 1/2 cup guacamole with 8 chips

Spicy Edamame

Ingredients:

- 2 cups edamame, shelled

- 1 tablespoon olive oil

- 1 teaspoon chili powder

- 1/2 teaspoon garlic powder

- Salt to taste

Instructions:

1. Steam or boil edamame until tender.
2. In a pan, heat olive oil, add edamame, chili powder, and garlic powder.
3. Sauté for 3-5 minutes, stirring frequently.
4. Sprinkle with salt and serve hot.

Nutrition Information (per serving):

- Calories: 120
- Protein: 11g
- Carbohydrates: 8g
- Fat: 5g
- Sodium: 5mg
- Potassium: 340mg
- Phosphorus: 120mg
- Portion Size: 1 cup edamame

Cucumber and Tomato Salsa

Ingredients:

- 1 cucumber, diced
- 2 tomatoes, diced
- 1/4 cup red onion, finely chopped
- 1 jalapeño, seeded and minced
- 2 tablespoons fresh cilantro, chopped
- 1 lime, juiced
- Salt and pepper to taste

Instructions:

1. In a bowl, combine diced cucumber, tomatoes, red onion, jalapeño, and cilantro.
2. Squeeze lime juice over the mixture and toss gently.
3. Season with salt and pepper to taste.
4. Chill in the refrigerator before serving.

Nutrition Information (per serving):

- Calories: 45
- Protein: 1g
- Carbohydrates: 10g
- Fat: 0.5g
- Sodium: 5mg
- Potassium: 280mg
- Phosphorus: 25mg
- Portion Size: 1/2 cup salsa

Vegan Spinach and Artichoke Dip

Ingredients:

- 1 cup frozen chopped spinach, thawed and drained
- 1 can (14 oz) artichoke hearts, drained and chopped
- 1 cup vegan cream cheese

- 1/2 cup vegan mayonnaise

- 1/2 cup nutritional yeast

- 2 cloves garlic, minced

- Salt and pepper to taste

- Whole grain pita bread for dipping

Instructions:

1. Preheat the oven to 350°F (175°C).

2. In a bowl, mix together spinach, artichoke hearts, vegan cream cheese, vegan mayonnaise, nutritional yeast, and minced garlic.

3. Season with salt and pepper to taste.

4. Transfer the mixture to a baking dish and bake for 25-30 minutes until bubbly.

5. Serve with whole grain pita bread.

Nutrition Information (per serving):

- Calories: 180

- Protein: 5g

- Carbohydrates: 12g

- Fat: 14g

- Sodium: 280mg

- Potassium: 200mg

- Phosphorus: 60mg

- Portion Size: 1/4 cup dip with 2 pieces of pita bread

Crispy Chickpeas with Smoky Paprika

Ingredients:

- 2 cans (15 oz each) chickpeas, drained and rinsed

- 2 tablespoons olive oil

- 1 teaspoon smoked paprika

- 1/2 teaspoon garlic powder

- 1/2 teaspoon cumin

- Salt to taste

Instructions:

1. Preheat the oven to 400°F (200°C).

2. Pat chickpeas dry, toss with olive oil, smoked paprika, garlic powder, cumin, and salt.

3. Spread on a baking sheet in a single layer.

4. Bake for 30-40 minutes until crispy, shaking the pan occasionally.

5. Cool before serving.

Nutrition Information (per serving):

- Calories: 140
- Protein: 6g
- Carbohydrates: 22g
- Fat: 4g
- Sodium: 150mg
- Potassium: 180mg
- Phosphorus: 120mg
- Portion Size: 1/2 cup chickpeas

Stuffed Grape Leaves with Quinoa

Ingredients:

- 1 jar grape leaves, drained
- 1 cup cooked quinoa
- 1/4 cup pine nuts, toasted
- 2 tablespoons fresh mint, chopped
- 2 tablespoons fresh dill, chopped
- 1 tablespoon lemon juice
- Salt and pepper to taste

Instructions:

1. In a bowl, mix cooked quinoa, toasted pine nuts, chopped mint, chopped dill, and lemon juice.
2. Lay out grape leaves, place a spoonful of the quinoa mixture in the center, and fold to create a small roll.
3. Steam for 15-20 minutes.
4. Serve warm or chilled.

Nutrition Information (per serving):

- Calories: 80
- Protein: 2g
- Carbohydrates: 14g
- Fat: 2g
- Sodium: 250mg
- Potassium: 60mg
- Phosphorus: 50mg
- Portion Size: 3 stuffed grape leaves

Vegan Caprese Skewers

Ingredients:

- 1 pint cherry tomatoes
- 1 package (8 oz) vegan mozzarella, cubed

- Fresh basil leaves
- Balsamic glaze for drizzling

Instructions:

1. Thread a tomato, a cube of vegan mozzarella, and a basil leaf onto small skewers.
2. Arrange on a serving platter.
3. Drizzle with balsamic glaze just before serving.

Nutrition Information (per serving):

- Calories: 120
- Protein: 5g
- Carbohydrates: 5g
- Fat: 8g
- Sodium: 180mg
- Potassium: 150mg
- Phosphorus: 70mg
- Portion Size: 4 skewers

Sweet Potato Fries with Garlic Aioli

Ingredients:

- 2 large sweet potatoes, cut into fries

- 2 tablespoons olive oil
- 1 teaspoon paprika
- 1/2 teaspoon garlic powder
- Salt and pepper to taste

For Garlic Aioli:
- 1/2 cup vegan mayonnaise
- 2 cloves garlic, minced
- 1 tablespoon lemon juice
- Salt and pepper to taste

Instructions:

1. Preheat the oven to 425°F (220°C).
2. Toss sweet potato fries with olive oil, paprika, garlic powder, salt, and pepper.
3. Spread on a baking sheet and bake for 25-30 minutes, turning halfway.
4. Mix garlic aioli ingredients in a bowl.
5. Serve sweet potato fries with garlic aioli.

Nutrition Information (per serving):
- Calories: 180

- Protein: 2g

- Carbohydrates: 20g

- Fat: 10g

- Sodium: 180mg

- Potassium: 320mg

- Phosphorus: 50mg

- Portion Size: 1 cup fries with 2 tablespoons aioli

Vegan Buffalo Cauliflower Bites

Ingredients:

- 1 head cauliflower, cut into florets

- 1/2 cup whole wheat flour

- 1/2 cup almond milk

- 1 teaspoon garlic powder

- 1 teaspoon onion powder

- 1/2 cup buffalo sauce

- 1 tablespoon vegan butter, melted

Instructions:

1. Preheat the oven to 450°F (230°C).

2. In a bowl, whisk together flour, almond milk, garlic powder, and onion powder to create a batter.

3. Dip cauliflower florets into the batter, ensuring they are well-coated, and place on a baking sheet.

4. Bake for 20 minutes, turning halfway.

5. In a separate bowl, mix buffalo sauce and melted vegan butter.

6. Toss baked cauliflower in the buffalo sauce mixture.

7. Bake for an additional 10 minutes.

8. Serve hot.

Nutrition Information (per serving):

- Calories: 120
- Protein: 4g
- Carbohydrates: 18g
- Fat: 4g
- Sodium: 520mg
- Potassium: 430mg
- Phosphorus: 70mg
- Portion Size: 1 cup cauliflower bites

Avocado and Black Bean Salsa

Ingredients:

- 2 ripe avocados, diced

- 1 can (15 oz) black beans, drained and rinsed
- 1 cup corn kernels (fresh or frozen)
- 1/4 cup red onion, finely chopped
- 1/4 cup fresh cilantro, chopped
- 1 lime, juiced
- Salt and pepper to taste

Instructions:

1. In a bowl, combine diced avocados, black beans, corn, red onion, cilantro, and lime juice.
2. Mix gently and season with salt and pepper to taste.
3. Chill in the refrigerator before serving.

Nutrition Information (per serving):

- Calories: 150
- Protein: 5g
- Carbohydrates: 22g
- Fat: 6g
- Sodium: 180mg
- Potassium: 480mg
- Phosphorus: 90mg
- Portion Size: 1/2 cup salsa

Vegan Pesto and Tomato Bruschetta

Ingredients:

- 1 baguette, sliced
- 1 cup cherry tomatoes, halved
- 1/2 cup vegan pesto
- 2 tablespoons balsamic glaze
- Fresh basil leaves for garnish

Instructions:

1. Toast baguette slices in the oven or on a grill.
2. Spread each slice with vegan pesto.
3. Top with cherry tomatoes.
4. Drizzle with balsamic glaze and garnish with fresh basil leaves.

Nutrition Information (per serving):

- Calories: 120
- Protein: 3g
- Carbohydrates: 16g
- Fat: 5g
- Sodium: 220mg
- Potassium: 120mg

- Phosphorus: 50mg

- Portion Size: 2 bruschetta slices

Green Pea and Mint Hummus

Ingredients:

- 1 can (15 oz) green peas, drained

- 1/4 cup fresh mint leaves

- 2 tablespoons tahini

- 2 tablespoons lemon juice

- 1 clove garlic, minced

- 2 tablespoons olive oil

- Salt and pepper to taste

- Whole grain crackers for dipping

Instructions:

1. In a food processor, combine green peas, fresh mint, tahini, lemon juice, and minced garlic.

2. Blend until smooth, gradually adding olive oil.

3. Season with salt and pepper to taste.

4. Serve with whole grain crackers.

Nutrition Information (per serving):

- Calories: 90

- Protein: 3g

- Carbohydrates: 10g

- Fat: 5g

- Sodium: 110mg

- Potassium: 140mg

- Phosphorus: 70mg

- Portion Size: 2 tablespoons hummus with crackers

Vegan Spring Rolls with Peanut Dipping Sauce

Ingredients:

For Spring Rolls:

- Rice paper wrappers

- 1 cup vermicelli rice noodles, cooked

- 1 cup lettuce, shredded

- 1 cup cucumber, julienned

- 1 cup carrots, julienned

- Fresh mint leaves

- Fresh cilantro leaves

For Peanut Dipping Sauce:

- 1/4 cup peanut butter
- 2 tablespoons soy sauce
- 1 tablespoon maple syrup
- 1 clove garlic, minced
- 1 teaspoon sesame oil
- Water (as needed for thinning)

Instructions:

1. Dip rice paper wrappers in warm water until pliable.
2. Place a small amount of vermicelli noodles, lettuce, cucumber, carrots, mint, and cilantro on each wrapper.
3. Roll tightly, folding in the sides, to form spring rolls.
4. For the dipping sauce, whisk together peanut butter, soy sauce, maple syrup, minced garlic, and sesame oil. Thin with water as needed.
5. Serve spring rolls with peanut dipping sauce.

Nutrition Information (per serving):

- Calories: 180
- Protein: 5g

- Carbohydrates: 30g
- Fat: 6g
- Sodium: 280mg
- Potassium: 220mg
- Phosphorus: 80mg
- Portion Size: 2 spring rolls with dipping sauce

Zucchini and Carrot Fritters

Ingredients:

- 2 zucchinis, grated
- 2 carrots, grated
- 1/4 cup whole wheat flour
- 1/4 cup nutritional yeast
- 2 green onions, chopped
- 1 teaspoon baking powder
- Salt and pepper to taste
- 2 tablespoons olive oil (for frying)

Instructions:

1. In a bowl, combine grated zucchini, grated carrots, whole wheat flour, nutritional yeast, chopped green onions, baking powder, salt, and pepper.

2. Heat olive oil in a pan over medium heat.

3. Scoop spoonfuls of the mixture into the pan, flattening to form fritters.

4. Cook for 3-4 minutes on each side until golden brown.

5. Serve hot.

Nutrition Information (per serving):

- Calories: 120
- Protein: 4g
- Carbohydrates: 14g
- Fat: 6g
- Sodium: 180mg
- Potassium: 310mg
- Phosphorus: 80mg
- Portion Size: 2 fritters

Chapter 6: Desserts

In this chapter, we present a delightful array of vegan desserts that not only satisfy your sweet cravings but also align with kidney-friendly dietary considerations. Each recipe is thoughtfully curated to bring you flavors, textures, and, most importantly, a guilt-free experience.

Vegan Chocolate Avocado Mousse

Ingredients:

- 2 ripe avocados
- 1/2 cup cocoa powder
- 1/2 cup maple syrup
- 1 tsp vanilla extract
- Pinch of salt

Instructions:

1. Blend avocados until smooth.
2. Add cocoa powder, maple syrup, vanilla extract, and salt.
3. Blend until creamy.

4. Chill before serving.

Nutrition Information (per serving):

- Calories: 180
- Protein: 2g
- Carbohydrates: 20g
- Fat: 12g
- Sodium: 10mg
- Potassium: 350mg
- Phosphorus: 45mg
- Portion Size: 1/2 cup

Berry and Almond Tart

Ingredients:

- 1 cup almonds
- 1 cup mixed berries
- 1/4 cup maple syrup
- 1 tsp vanilla extract
- 1 tbsp lemon juice

Instructions:

1. Blend almonds into a crust.

2. Mix berries, maple syrup, vanilla, and lemon juice.

3. Fill the crust with the berry mixture.

4. Chill before serving.

Nutrition Information (per serving):

- Calories: 220

- Protein: 5g

- Carbohydrates: 18g

- Fat: 15g

- Sodium: 5mg

- Potassium: 180mg

- Phosphorus: 65mg

- Portion Size: 1 slice

Vegan Pumpkin Pie

Ingredients:

- 1 can pumpkin puree

- 1/2 cup coconut milk

- 1/2 cup maple syrup

- 1 tsp pumpkin spice

- 1 prepared vegan pie crust

Instructions:

1. Mix pumpkin, coconut milk, maple syrup, and spice.

2. Pour into the pie crust.

3. Bake until set.

Nutrition Information (per serving):

- Calories: 250

- Protein: 3g

- Carbohydrates: 28g

- Fat: 15g

- Sodium: 180mg

- Potassium: 220mg

- Phosphorus: 50mg

- Portion Size: 1 slice

Coconut and Mango Sorbet

Ingredients:

- 2 cups mango, frozen

- 1 can coconut milk

- 1/4 cup agave syrup

- 1 tbsp lime juice

Instructions:

1. Blend mango, coconut milk, agave, and lime juice.
2. Freeze until firm.

Nutrition Information (per serving):

- Calories: 180
- Protein: 2g
- Carbohydrates: 25g
- Fat: 9g
- Sodium: 20mg
- Potassium: 240mg
- Phosphorus: 30mg
- Portion Size: 1/2 cup

Vegan Lemon Blueberry Cheesecake

Ingredients:

- 2 cups cashews, soaked
- 1/2 cup coconut oil
- 1/2 cup maple syrup
- Zest and juice of 2 lemons
- 1 cup blueberries

Instructions:

1. Blend cashews, coconut oil, maple syrup, lemon zest, and juice.
2. Pour over a crust and top with blueberries.
3. Chill before serving.

Nutrition Information (per serving):

- Calories: 280
- Protein: 6g
- Carbohydrates: 22g
- Fat: 20g
- Sodium: 10mg
- Potassium: 220mg
- Phosphorus: 70mg
- Portion Size: 1 slice

Chocolate-Dipped Strawberries

Ingredients:

- 1 cup dark chocolate chips
- 16 fresh strawberries

Instructions:

1. Melt chocolate in a bowl.
2. Dip strawberries in melted chocolate.
3. Place on parchment paper to set.

Nutrition Information (per serving):

- Calories: 120
- Protein: 2g
- Carbohydrates: 15g
- Fat: 7g
- Sodium: 5mg
- Potassium: 150mg
- Phosphorus: 30mg
- Portion Size: 4 strawberries

Vegan Banana Bread Pudding

Ingredients:

- 4 ripe bananas
- 4 cups cubed whole grain bread
- 2 cups almond milk
- 1/2 cup maple syrup
- 1 tsp cinnamon

Instructions:

1. Mash bananas and mix with bread cubes.
2. Combine almond milk, maple syrup, and cinnamon.
3. Pour over the bread mixture.
4. Bake until golden.

Nutrition Information (per serving):

- Calories: 220
- Protein: 5g
- Carbohydrates: 40g
- Fat: 4g
- Sodium: 180mg
- Potassium: 350mg
- Phosphorus: 80mg
- Portion Size: 1 cup

Almond and Raspberry Thumbprint Cookies

Ingredients:

- 1 cup almond flour
- 1/4 cup coconut oil

- 1/4 cup maple syrup
- 1/2 cup raspberry jam

Instructions:

1. Mix almond flour, coconut oil, and maple syrup.
2. Form cookies, make a thumbprint, and fill with jam.
3. Bake until golden.

Nutrition Information (per serving):

- Calories: 160
- Protein: 3g
- Carbohydrates: 14g
- Fat: 10g
- Sodium: 5mg
- Potassium: 90mg
- Phosphorus: 40mg
- Portion Size: 2 cookies

Vegan Apple Crisp

Ingredients:

- 4 apples, sliced
- 1 cup rolled oats

- 1/2 cup almond flour

- 1/4 cup maple syrup

- 1 tsp cinnamon

Instructions:

1. Mix apples with maple syrup and cinnamon.

2. Combine oats and almond flour.

3. Top apples with oat mixture.

4. Bake until apples are tender.

Nutrition Information (per serving):

- Calories: 180

- Protein: 4g

- Carbohydrates: 32g

- Fat: 5g

- Sodium: 5mg

- Potassium: 200mg

- Phosphorus: 60mg

- Portion Size: 1 cup

Avocado Lime Vegan Cheesecake Bars

Ingredients:

- 2 avocados
- 1 cup almonds
- 1/4 cup coconut oil
- 1/2 cup lime juice
- 1/2 cup agave syrup

Instructions:

1. Blend avocados, almonds, coconut oil, lime juice, and agave.
2. Press into a pan and chill until set.

Nutrition Information (per serving):

- Calories: 220
- Protein: 4g
- Carbohydrates: 18g
- Fat: 15g
- Sodium: 5mg
- Potassium: 300mg
- Phosphorus: 70mg

- Portion Size: 1 bar

Chocolate Peanut Butter Energy Bites

Ingredients:

- 1 cup rolled oats
- 1/2 cup peanut butter
- 1/4 cup cocoa powder
- 1/4 cup maple syrup
- 1 tsp vanilla extract

Instructions:

1. Mix oats, peanut butter, cocoa powder, maple syrup, and vanilla.
2. Form into bite-sized balls.
3. Chill before serving.

Nutrition Information (per serving):

- Calories: 160
- Protein: 5g
- Carbohydrates: 18g

- Fat: 8g

- Sodium: 40mg

- Potassium: 150mg

- Phosphorus: 60mg

- Portion Size: 2 bites

Vegan Carrot Cake with Cashew Cream Frosting

Ingredients:

- 2 cups shredded carrots

- 1 cup whole wheat flour

- 1/2 cup almond flour

- 1/2 cup coconut oil

- 1/2 cup maple syrup

- 1 tsp cinnamon

Instructions:

1. Mix carrots, whole wheat flour, almond flour, coconut oil, maple syrup, and cinnamon.

2. Bake until golden.

3. Frost with cashew cream.

Nutrition Information (per serving):

- Calories: 240
- Protein: 4g
- Carbohydrates: 25g
- Fat: 15g
- Sodium: 30mg
- Potassium: 280mg
- Phosphorus: 70mg
- Portion Size: 1 slice

Blueberry Coconut Bliss Balls

Ingredients:

- 1 cup dried blueberries
- 1 cup shredded coconut
- 1/2 cup almonds
- 1/4 cup maple syrup
- 1 tsp vanilla extract

Instructions:

1. Blend blueberries, coconut, almonds, maple syrup, and vanilla.
2. Form into small balls.

3. Refrigerate until firm.

Nutrition Information (per serving):

- Calories: 180

- Protein: 3g

- Carbohydrates: 22g

- Fat: 10g

- Sodium: 5mg

- Potassium: 160mg

- Phosphorus: 40mg

- Portion Size: 2 balls

Vegan Peach Cobbler

Ingredients:

- 4 cups sliced peaches

- 1 cup rolled oats

- 1/2 cup almond flour

- 1/4 cup maple syrup

- 1 tsp vanilla extract

Instructions:

1. Mix peaches, rolled oats, almond flour, maple syrup, and vanilla.

2. Bake until peaches are bubbly.

Nutrition Information (per serving):

- Calories: 200
- Protein: 4g
- Carbohydrates: 30g
- Fat: 8g
- Sodium: 5mg
- Potassium: 220mg
- Phosphorus: 60mg
- Portion Size: 1 cup

Dark Chocolate Avocado Truffles

Ingredients:

- 2 ripe avocados
- 1/2 cup dark chocolate, melted
- 1/4 cup cocoa powder
- 1/4 cup powdered sugar
- 1 tsp vanilla extract

Instructions:

1. Blend avocados until smooth.
2. Add melted chocolate, cocoa powder, powdered sugar, and vanilla.
3. Form into truffles and chill.

Nutrition Information (per serving):

- Calories: 180
- Protein: 2g
- Carbohydrates: 16g
- Fat: 12g
- Sodium: 5mg
- Potassium: 270mg
- Phosphorus: 50mg
- Portion Size: 2 truffles

Chapter 7: Smoothies

These delightful concoctions not only tantalize your taste buds but also contribute to your well-being. Packed with essential vitamins and minerals, these smoothies are a testament to the fusion of flavors and health benefits.

Green Detox Smoothie

Ingredients:

- 1 cup kale, stems removed
- 1 green apple, cored and chopped
- 1 cucumber, peeled and sliced
- 1 lemon, juiced
- 1 cup coconut water
- Ice cubes (optional)

Instructions:

1. Blend kale, green apple, cucumber, and lemon juice until smooth.
2. Add coconut water and blend again until well combined.

3. If desired, add ice cubes and blend until the desired consistency is reached.

Nutrition Information:

- Calories: 120
- Protein: 3g
- Carbohydrates: 28g
- Fat: 1g
- Sodium: 50mg
- Potassium: 550mg
- Phosphorus: 80mg
- Portion Size: 1 serving

Berry Blast Smoothie

Ingredients:

- 1 cup mixed berries (strawberries, blueberries, raspberries)
- 1 banana, peeled
- 1/2 cup almond milk
- 1 tablespoon chia seeds
- Honey or agave syrup to taste
- Ice cubes (optional)

Instructions:

1. Combine mixed berries, banana, almond milk, and chia seeds in a blender.

2. Add honey or agave syrup to taste.

3. Blend until smooth and creamy.

4. For a colder version, add ice cubes and blend again.

Nutrition Information:

- Calories: 150

- Protein: 4g

- Carbohydrates: 35g

- Fat: 2g

- Sodium: 30mg

- Potassium: 300mg

- Phosphorus: 90mg

- Portion Size: 1 serving

Tropical Turmeric Smoothie

Ingredients:

- 1 cup pineapple chunks

- 1/2 mango, peeled and diced

- 1 teaspoon turmeric powder

- 1 tablespoon flaxseeds

- 1 cup coconut water

- Ice cubes (optional)

Instructions:

1. Blend pineapple, mango, turmeric powder, and flaxseeds until smooth.

2. Add coconut water and blend until well mixed.

3. Optionally, include ice cubes for a chilled experience.

Nutrition Information:

- Calories: 140

- Protein: 3.5g

- Carbohydrates: 32g

- Fat: 2g

- Sodium: 40mg

- Potassium: 450mg

- Phosphorus: 70mg

- Portion Size: 1 serving

Kale and Pineapple Smoothie

Ingredients:

- 2 cups kale, stems removed
- 1 cup pineapple chunks
- 1 banana, peeled
- 1/2 cup coconut milk
- 1 tablespoon hemp seeds
- Ice cubes (optional)

Instructions:

1. Blend kale, pineapple, banana, coconut milk, and hemp seeds until smooth.
2. Add ice cubes and blend for a refreshing texture.

Nutrition Information:

- Calories: 130
- Protein: 5g
- Carbohydrates: 28g
- Fat: 2.5g
- Sodium: 25mg
- Potassium: 470mg
- Phosphorus: 100mg

- Portion Size: 1 serving

Mango and Coconut Smoothie

Ingredients:

- 1 cup ripe mango, diced
- 1/2 cup coconut milk
- 1/2 cup water
- 1 tablespoon shredded coconut
- 1 teaspoon lime juice
- Ice cubes (optional)

Instructions:

1. Blend ripe mango, coconut milk, water, shredded coconut, and lime juice until smooth.
2. Add ice cubes if desired, and blend until well incorporated.

Nutrition Information:

- Calories: 160
- Protein: 2g
- Carbohydrates: 35g
- Fat: 4g

- Sodium: 15mg

- Potassium: 380mg

- Phosphorus: 60mg

- Portion Size: 1 serving

Spinach and Banana Smoothie

Ingredients:

- 2 cups fresh spinach

- 2 ripe bananas, peeled

- 1/2 cup almond milk

- 1 tablespoon peanut butter

- 1 teaspoon honey (optional)

- Ice cubes (optional)

Instructions:

1. Blend fresh spinach, ripe bananas, almond milk, peanut butter, and honey until smooth.

2. Add ice cubes for a cooler consistency.

Nutrition Information:

- Calories: 180

- Protein: 5g

- Carbohydrates: 32g

- Fat: 6g

- Sodium: 80mg

- Potassium: 700mg

- Phosphorus: 120mg

- Portion Size: 1 serving

Blueberry Almond Butter Smoothie

Ingredients:

- 1 cup blueberries

- 1 banana, peeled

- 2 tablespoons almond butter

- 1/2 cup almond milk

- 1 tablespoon flaxseeds

- Ice cubes (optional)

Instructions:

1. Blend blueberries, banana, almond butter, almond milk, and flaxseeds until smooth.

2. Incorporate ice cubes for added freshness.

Nutrition Information:

- Calories: 200
- Protein: 5g
- Carbohydrates: 35g
- Fat: 7g
- Sodium: 40mg
- Potassium: 380mg
- Phosphorus: 100mg
- Portion Size: 1 serving

Beet and Berry Power Smoothie

Ingredients:

- 1 small beet, peeled and diced
- 1/2 cup mixed berries (strawberries, raspberries, blueberries)
- 1/2 cup orange juice
- 1 tablespoon chia seeds
- 1/2 cup water
- Ice cubes (optional)

Instructions:

1. Blend beet, mixed berries, orange juice, chia seeds, and water until smooth.

2. For a chilled version, include ice cubes in the blending process.

Nutrition Information:

- Calories: 160
- Protein: 3g
- Carbohydrates: 35g
- Fat: 2g
- Sodium: 20mg
- Potassium: 400mg
- Phosphorus: 80mg
- Portion Size: 1 serving

Orange Creamsicle Smoothie

Ingredients:

- 1 cup orange segments
- 1 frozen banana, peeled
- 1/2 cup vanilla almond milk
- 1 tablespoon coconut cream

- 1 teaspoon agave syrup
- Ice cubes (optional)

Instructions:

1. Blend orange segments, frozen banana, vanilla almond milk, coconut cream, and agave syrup until creamy.
2. Add ice cubes for a frosty texture.

Nutrition Information:

- Calories: 150
- Protein: 2.5g
- Carbohydrates: 30g
- Fat: 3.5g
- Sodium: 25mg
- Potassium: 380mg
- Phosphorus: 70mg
- Portion Size: 1 serving

Avocado and Mint Smoothie

Ingredients:

- 1 ripe avocado, peeled and pitted

- 1/2 cup fresh mint leaves
- 1/2 cup spinach
- 1 tablespoon lime juice
- 1 cup coconut water
- Ice cubes (optional)

Instructions:

1. Blend ripe avocado, fresh mint leaves, spinach, lime juice, and coconut water until smooth.
2. Include ice cubes for a chilled experience.

Nutrition Information:

- Calories: 170
- Protein: 3g
- Carbohydrates: 30g
- Fat: 6g
- Sodium: 45mg
- Potassium: 600mg
- Phosphorus: 90mg
- Portion Size: 1 serving

Chia Seed and Mixed Berry Smoothie

Ingredients:

- 1/4 cup chia seeds
- 1 cup mixed berries (strawberries, blueberries, raspberries)
- 1 banana, peeled
- 1 cup almond milk
- 1 tablespoon honey
- Ice cubes (optional)

Instructions:

1. Soak chia seeds in almond milk for 10 minutes until they form a gel-like consistency.
2. Blend soaked chia seeds, mixed berries, banana, and honey until smooth.
3. Add ice cubes for a refreshing twist.

Nutrition Information:

- Calories: 180
- Protein: 5g
- Carbohydrates: 30g

- Fat: 6g

- Sodium: 35mg

- Potassium: 400mg

- Phosphorus: 80mg

- Portion Size: 1 serving

Protein-Packed Peanut Butter Smoothie

Ingredients:

- 2 tablespoons peanut butter

- 1 banana, peeled

- 1/2 cup oats

- 1 cup almond milk

- 1 teaspoon honey (optional)

- Ice cubes (optional)

Instructions:

1. Blend peanut butter, banana, oats, almond milk, and honey until smooth.

2. For added freshness, include ice cubes in the blending process.

Nutrition Information:

- Calories: 250
- Protein: 8g
- Carbohydrates: 35g
- Fat: 9g
- Sodium: 80mg
- Potassium: 500mg
- Phosphorus: 120mg
- Portion Size: 1 serving

Papaya and Lime Smoothie

Ingredients:

- 1 cup ripe papaya, diced
- 1/2 cup pineapple chunks
- 1 tablespoon lime juice
- 1/2 cup coconut water
- 1 tablespoon chia seeds
- Ice cubes (optional)

Instructions:

1. Blend ripe papaya, pineapple chunks, lime juice, coconut water, and chia seeds until smooth.

2. If a colder drink is preferred, add ice cubes during
   blending.

Nutrition Information:

- Calories: 140
- Protein: 2.5g
- Carbohydrates: 30g
- Fat: 3g
- Sodium: 20mg
- Potassium: 450mg
- Phosphorus: 80mg
- Portion Size: 1 serving

Cucumber and Kiwi Cooler

Ingredients:

- 1 cucumber, peeled and sliced
- 2 kiwis, peeled and chopped
- 1/2 cup mint leaves
- 1 tablespoon lime juice
- 1 cup coconut water
- Ice cubes (optional)

Instructions:

1. Blend cucumber, kiwis, mint leaves, lime juice, and coconut water until well combined.

2. Enhance the freshness by adding ice cubes during blending.

Nutrition Information:

- Calories: 120

- Protein: 2g

- Carbohydrates: 25g

- Fat: 2g

- Sodium: 30mg

- Potassium: 380mg

- Phosphorus: 60mg

- Portion Size: 1 serving

Chocolate Avocado Protein Smoothie

Ingredients:

- 1 ripe avocado, peeled and pitted

- 2 tablespoons cocoa powder

- 1 scoop plant-based protein powder
- 1 cup almond milk
- 1 tablespoon maple syrup
- Ice cubes (optional)

Instructions:

1. Blend ripe avocado, cocoa powder, plant-based protein powder, almond milk, and maple syrup until smooth.
2. For an extra chill, incorporate ice cubes during blending.

Nutrition Information:

- Calories: 230
- Protein: 12g
- Carbohydrates: 25g
- Fat: 10g
- Sodium: 60mg
- Potassium: 580mg
- Phosphorus: 100mg
- Portion Size: 1 serving

CONCLUSION

As we reach the end of this kidney-friendly vegan culinary expedition, it's not merely the conclusion of a cookbook, but the commencement of a transformative gastronomic journey. "Nourishing Roots: A Kidney-Friendly Vegan Cookbook" stands as a testament to the harmonious blend of health-conscious choices and delectable flavors, ensuring that your dietary path to kidney wellness is paved with culinary delight.

In this collection, we've not just assembled recipes; we've curated an experience—an exploration of the vibrant world of plant-based ingredients that not only cater to kidney health but elevate your taste buds to new heights. Each chapter, a chapter in your personal wellness story, is crafted with precision and passion, offering a diverse array of breakfasts, lunches, dinners, snacks, desserts, and smoothies.

From the wholesome 30-day meal plan designed for simplicity and variety to the tantalizing smoothies that refresh and revitalize, every page resonates with the philosophy that good food should not only sustain the body but also feed the soul. The recipes aren't just a collection; they are an invitation to savor the symphony of flavors derived from nature's bounty.

As you embark on this culinary expedition, may you discover the joy in preparing meals that nourish and nurture. The cookbook is a guide, a companion on your kitchen counter, encouraging you to explore, experiment, and enjoy the process of creating wholesome, kidney-friendly masterpieces.

Remember, this isn't just about the recipes; it's about embracing a lifestyle that supports your well-being. Each dish is a celebration of the intricate dance between health-conscious choices and the pleasure of eating. It's a testament to the idea that taking care of our bodies can be a delightful and fulfilling experience.

So, here's to a journey of wellness, one delicious plate at a time. May your kitchen be filled with the aromas of compassion, health, and joy. "Nourishing Roots" isn't just a cookbook; it's a culinary companion, guiding you towards a healthier, tastier, and more fulfilling way of life.

Bon appétit and here's to your vibrant health!